EASY TO PREPARE DIABETIC COOKBOOK

50 SIMPLE AND EASY RECIPES FOR NUTRITIONALLY BALANCED MEALS

Table of Contents

INTRODUCTION 4

RECIPES 6

- BREAKFAST 6
    - 1 Gingerbread Oatmeal 6
    - 2 Assorted Fresh Fruit Juice 7
    - 3 Raspberry and Pineapple Smoothie (Dairy-Free) 7
    - 4 Mexican Frittata 8
    - 5 Olive Oil and Sesame Asparagus 9
    - 6 Tuna Salad 10
    - 7 Quinoa Congee with Cauliflower 11
- GRAINS 12
    - 8 Chickpea Tortillas 12
    - 9 "Cornbread" Stuffing 13
    - 10 "Flour" Tortillas 15
    - 11 Flourless "Burger Buns" 16
    - 12 Fried Rice 17
    - 13 Garlic Basil Breadsticks 17
- SEAFOOD 19
    - 14 Grilled Tuna Salad 19
    - 15 Crab Curry 20
    - 16 Mussels And Spaghetti Squash 21
    - 17 Shrimp With Tomatoes And Feta 22
    - 18 Lemon Pepper And Dill Salmon 23
- POULTRY 25
    - 19 Chicken With Cashew Nuts 25
    - 20 Chuck And Veggies 26
    - 21 Chicken & Broccoli Bake 27
    - 22 Hoisin Chicken Lettuce Wraps 28
    - 23 Zucchini With Tomatoes 30
    - 24 Chicken Liver Curry 31
- SOUP AND STEWS 32
    - 25 Chipotle Chicken & Corn Soup 32
    - 26 Chorizo & Corn Chowder 33
    - 27 Chunky Chicken Noodle Soup 34
    - 28 Cioppino 36
    - 29 Clam & Bacon Soup 38
    - 30 Crab & Cauliflower Bisque 39
    - 31 Creamy Chicken & Cauliflower Rice Soup 40
    - 32 Creamy Sweet Potato & Cauliflower Bisque 42
    - 33 Curried Chicken Soup 43

SALADS, SAUCES, DRESSINGS & DIPS   44
- 34 Parmesan-Topped Acorn Squash   44
- 35 Quinoa Tabbouleh   46
- 36 Wild Rice Salad with Cranberries and Almonds   47
- 37 Low Fat Roasties   49

DESSERT AND SNACKS   50
- 38 Green Fruity Smoothie   50
- 39 Baked Creamy Custard With Maple   51
- 40 Lemon Cookies   52
- 41 Pineapple Nice Cream   53
- 42 Garden Salad Wraps   54
- 43 Berry Mint Smoothie   55
- 44 Greenie Smoothie   56
- 45 Coconut Spinach Smoothie   57
- 46 Oats Coffee Smoothie   58
- 47 Avocado Smoothie   59
- 48 Orange Carrot Smoothie   60
- 49 Blackberry Smoothie   60
- 50 Key Lime Pie Smoothie   61

CONCLUSION   62

Introduction

Diabetes is a condition where the body is no longer able to self-regulate blood glucose. When you eat a food that contains carbohydrate—whether it comes from honey, an apple, or brown rice—the body breaks it down into sugar (also called glucose) during digestion. This glucose passes through the walls of the intestines into the blood, which causes blood sugar (the amount of glucose circulating in the blood) to rise. In response, the pancreas secretes a hormone called insulin. The role of insulin is to lower the blood sugar back to normal levels. It does this by moving the sugar out of the blood and into the cells, where it is used for energy. Think of insulin as a key that unlocks the doors to the cells. But if you have diabetes, either the body doesn't make enough insulin or the cells don't respond to the insulin. This causes the blood sugar to build up in the bloodstream, resulting in high blood sugar. Type 2 diabetes usually begins with insulin resistance. The muscle, fat, and liver cells no longer respond to insulin, so the pancreas secretes large amounts of it, trying to keep blood sugar levels within a normal range. Being overweight and physically inactive contributes further to insulin resistance. Insulin resistance is also found in prediabetes or glucose intolerance. An estimated 79 million Americans have prediabetes. I tell my patients that prediabetes is a warning bell to take action to help prevent diabetes. Studies have shown that losing 7 percent of your body weight, along with regular exercise, can decrease the risk of type 2 diabetes by 58 percent. Once you have diabetes, losing weight, regular exercise, eating carbohydrates in moderation, and maintaining a healthy diet can decrease insulin resistance. This, in turn, will promote better blood sugar control.

A diabetes diagnosis means that the pancreas is not able to produce enough insulin to keep up with this resistance—and insulin deficiency is the result. If your body can't make enough insulin, blood sugar levels become elevated. Long-term elevated blood sugar levels can affect almost every system in the body. Health complications can include heart disease, stroke, kidney failure, nerve damage, eye damage, and blindness. This is why it is so important to work with your health-care team to come up with the best treatment plan for you, and for you to take the leading part in your plan by eating healthy, staying physically active, and losing weight if necessary.

According to the CDC, there are more than 30 million individuals in America that have diabetes; and 1 in 4 of these people don't know they have this condition. The cause of diabetes is linked with the pancreases, which fail to produce or use insulin properly. Insulin hormone is secreted into the bloodstream by the pancreatic gland to deliver it into the cells. Once, the cells take in the sugar, it is then converted into energy and use immediately or store for later use.

The link between obesity and type 2 Diabetes

Although the exact cause of type 2 diabetes is still not fully understood, being obese and overweight is believed to account 80 percent of the risk of developing diabetes. So, if you have excess weight around your tummy, you are at greater risk of developing type 2 diabetes. In obese people, the abdominal fat cells have to more nutrients than average, and then this stress in the cell makes them release pro-inflammatory chemicals. These chemicals disrupt the function of insulin hormone and/or makes the body less sensitive to the insulin. This is known as insulin resistance which is the major cause of type 2 diabetes. Therefore, having excess abdominal fat or large waistline leads to high risk of diabetes.

Recipes

Breakfast

1 Gingerbread Oatmeal

Preparation time: 10 minutes

Cooking time: 15 minutes

Servings: 4

Ingredients:

1 cup steel cut oats

4 cups water

¼ teaspoon ground coriander

1½ tablespoons ground cinnamon

¼ teaspoon ground cloves

¼ teaspoon fresh grated ginger

¼ teaspoon ground allspice

¼ teaspoon ground cardamom

A pinch of ground nutmeg

Directions:

Heat up a pan with the water over medium-high heat, add the oats and stir. Add the coriander, cinnamon, cloves, ginger, allspice, cardamom and nutmeg, stir, cook for 15 minutes, divide into bowls and serve.

Enjoy!

Nutrition: calories 188, fat 3, fiber 6, carbs 13, protein 6

2 Assorted Fresh Fruit Juice

Preparation time: 5 minutes

Cooking time:0 minutes

Servings:4

Ingredients:

1 cup ice shavings or crushed ice

¼ cup frozen grapes, halved

1 apple, roughly chopped

Directions:

Add all ingredients into blender.

Process until smooth.

Pour equal portions into glasses. Serve immediately.

Nutrition: Protein 1.16g (2%), Potassium (K) 367 mg (8 %) and Sodium, Na 3 mg (0%)

3 Raspberry and Pineapple Smoothie (Dairy-Free)

Preparation time: 5 minutes

Cooking time:0 minutes

Servings:4

Ingredients:

1 can, 8 oz, pineapple tidbits, rinsed well, drained

1-piece, small overripe banana, roughly chopped

½ cup frozen raspberries

½ cup crushed ice

Directions:

Except for cashew nuts and stevia, combine remaining ingredients in a deep microwave-safe bowl. Stir.

Microwave on highest setting for 5 to 15 seconds. Keep a watchful eye on this. Stop the cooking process before milk bubbles out of the bowl.

Carefully remove bowl from microwave. Cool slightly for easier handling.

Stir in stevia if using. Sprinkle cashew nuts.

Nutrition: Protein 3.1g (6%), Potassium (K) 749 mg (16 %) and Sodium, Na 4 mg (0%)

4 Mexican Frittata

Preparation time: 5 minutes

Cooking time:30 minutes

Servings:4

Ingredients:

½ cup almond milk

5 large eggs

¼ cup onions, chopped

¼ cup green bell pepper, chopped

Directions:

Preheat the oven to 400° F.

Using a large bowl, combine almond milk, eggs, onion, and green bell pepper. Whisk until all ingredients are well combined.

Transfer the mixture to a baking dish. Bake for 20 minutes. Serve.

Nutrition: Protein 16.35g (30%), Potassium (K) 243 mg (5 %) and Sodium, Na 216 mg (14%)

5   Olive Oil and Sesame Asparagus

Preparation time: 5 minutes

Cooking time:30 minutes

Servings:4

Ingredients:

½ cup water

2 cups asparagus, sliced

½ tablespoon olive oil, add more for drizzling

1/8 teaspoon red pepper flakes, crushed

½ teaspoon sesame seeds

Directions:

In a large skillet, bring water to a boil.

Add in asparagus. Allow to boil for 2 minutes. Reduce the heat and cook for another 5 minutes. Drain asparagus and place on a plate. Set aside.

Meanwhile, heat the olive oil. Tip in asparagus and red pepper flakes. Saute for 3 minutes.

Remove from heat. Drizzle in more olive oil and sprinkle sesame seeds before serving.

Nutrition: Protein 6.19g (11%), Potassium (K) 547 mg (12 %) and Sodium, Na 9 mg (1%)

6 Tuna Salad

Preparation time: 5 minutes

Cooking time:10 minutes

Servings:4

Ingredients:

1 can of tuna, drained

1 cup onion, minced

1 celery, minced

Fresh herbs of choice

Directions:

In a salad bowl, put together salmon, mayonnaise, onion, pickle relish, celery, and fresh herbs of choice.

Mix all the ingredients until well combined. Serve.

Nutrition: Protein 21.89g (40%), Potassium (K) 284 mg (6 %) and Sodium, Na 222 mg (15%)

7 Quinoa Congee with Cauliflower

Preparation time: 5 minutes

Cooking time:20 minutes

Servings:4

Ingredients:

6 cups water

¼ cup quinoa

4 large leeks, minced, reserve green stems for garnish

1 small cauliflower head, minced

1 can mackerel in water, low-sodium, include liquid, flaked

1 tablespoon fresh ginger, grate

1 tablespoon low-sodium teriyaki sauce, add more later only if needed

¼ pound frozen scallops, thawed

½ pound frozen shrimps, thawed

Pinch of sea salt

Pinch of white pepper

1 lime, sliced into wedges

Directions:

Except for lime, scallops, and shrimps, pour remaining ingredients into slow cooker set at low heat. Stir. Put lid on. Cook for 6 hours. Stir in scallops and shrimps; cook for another 15 minutes. Turn off heat. Taste: adjust seasoning if needed.

Ladle congee into individual bowls. Garnish with leeks. Serve with wedge of lime on the side. Squeeze lime juice into congee just before eating.

Nutrition: Protein 10.11g (19%), Potassium (K) 364 mg (8 %) and Sodium, Na 180 mg (12%)

Grains

8 Chickpea Tortillas

Preparation time: 5 minutes
Cooking time: 10 minutes
Servings: 4
Ingredients:
1 cup chickpea flour
1 cup water
¼ tsp salt
Nonstick cooking spray
Directions:

In a large bowl, whisk all Ingredients together until no lumps remain.

Spray a skillet with cooking spray and place over med-high heat.

Pour batter in, ¼ cup at a time, and tilt pan to spread thinly.

Cook until golden brown on each side, about 2 minutes per side.

Use for taco shells, enchiladas, quesadillas or whatever you desire.

Nutrition:

Calories 89 Total Carbs 13g Net Carbs 10g Protein 5g Fat 2g Sugar 3g Fiber 3g

9 "Cornbread" Stuffing

Preparation time: 15 minutes

Cooking time: 40 minutes

Servings: 6

Ingredients:

1 strip bacon, diced

1 egg

1 cup onion, diced

1 cup celery, diced

2 tbsp. margarine, divided

What you'll need from store cupboard:

1 cup almond flour

¼ cup low sodium chicken broth

3 cloves garlic, diced fine

2 tbsp. stone-ground cornmeal

1 tsp thyme

1 tsp sage

¾ tsp salt

Fresh ground black pepper, to taste

Directions:

Heat the oven to 375 degrees.

Melt 1 tablespoon margarine in a skillet over low heat. Add onions and celery and cook, stirring, until soft, about 10 minutes. Add garlic and seasonings and cook 1-2 minutes more. Remove from heat and let cool.

Place the almond flour, cornmeal and bacon in a food processor and pulse until combined. Add the broth and egg and pulse just to combine. Add the onion mixture and pulse just until mixed.

Place remaining tablespoon of margarine in a cast iron skillet, or baking dish, and melt in the oven until hot. Swirl the pan to coat with melted margarine.

Spread the dressing in the pan and bake 30 minutes or until top is nicely browned and center is cooked through. Serve.

Nutrition:

Calories 177 Total Carbs 9g Net Carbs 6g Protein 6g Fat 14g Sugar 2g Fiber 3g

10 "Flour" Tortillas

Preparation time: 10 minutes

Cooking time 15 minutes

Servings: 4

Ingredients:

¾ cup egg whites

What you'll need from store cupboard:

1/3 cup water

¼ cup coconut flour

1 tsp sunflower oil

½ tsp salt

½ tsp cumin

½ tsp chili powder

Directions:

Add all Ingredients, except oil, to a food processor and pulse until combined. Let rest 7-8 minutes.

Heat oil in a large skillet over med-low heat. Pour ¼ cup batter into center and tilt to spread to 7-8-inch circle.

When the top is no longer shiny, flip tortilla and cook another 1-2 minutes. Repeat with remaining batter.

Place each tortilla on parchment paper and slightly wipe off any access oil.

Nutrition:

Calories 27 Total Carbs 1g Protein 5g Fat 0g Sugar 0g Fiber 0g

11   Flourless "Burger Buns"

Preparation time: 10 minutes

Cooking time: 35 minutes

Servings: 4

Ingredients:

4 egg yolks, room temp

4 egg whites, room temp

¼ cup low fat ricotta cheese

What you'll need from store cupboard:

¼ cup reduced fat parmesan cheese

1/4 tsp cream of tartar

Directions:

Heat oven to 300 degrees. Line a baking sheet with parchment paper.

In a large bowl, whisk egg yolks, ricotta and parmesan cheese until smooth.

In a separate bowl, beat egg whites until foamy, then add in cream of tartar and beat until stiff peaks form.

Add some beaten egg white to the egg yolk mixture and mix lightly. Slowly and lightly fold in the remaining egg white to the egg yolk mixture until just blended.

Spoon the batter onto prepared pan to make 8 buns. Bake 35 minutes. Use as bread for sandwiches or eat on its own.

Nutrition:

Calories 50 Total Carbs 1g Protein 4g Fat 3g Sugar 1g Fiber 0g

12   Fried Rice

Preparation time: 5 minutes

Cooking time: 15 minutes

Servings: 8

Ingredients:

2 cups sugar snap peas

2 egg whites

1 egg

What you'll need from store cupboard:

1 cup instant brown rice, cooked according to directions

2 tbsp. lite soy sauce

Directions:

Add the peas to the cooked rice and mix to combine.

In a small skillet, scramble the egg and egg whites. Add the rice and peas to the skillet and stir in soy sauce. Cook, stirring frequently, about 2-3 minutes, or until heated through. Serve.

Nutrition:

Calories 107 Total Carbs 20g Net Carbs 19g Protein 4g Fat 1g Sugar 1g Fiber 1g

13   Garlic Basil Breadsticks

Preparation time: 10 minutes

Cooking time: 10 minutes

Servings: 4

Ingredients:

2 eggs, beaten

2 cup mozzarella cheese, grated

2 tbsp. cream cheese

2 tbsp. fresh basil, diced

What you'll need from store cupboard:

4 tbsp. coconut flour

4 cloves garlic, crushed

Nonstick cooking spray

Directions:

Heat oven to 400 degrees. Spray a baking sheet with cooking spray.

Add mozzarella, cream cheese, crushed garlic and basil to a microwaveable bowl. Mix and then cook for 1 minute. Stir well to make sure the cheeses are melted and then add in the flour and egg.

Mix well, use your hands if needed to form into a dough. Break off pieces of the dough and roll into a long finger shapes. Place on prepared pan.

Bake 8-10 minutes or until the dough begins to brown. Remove from heat and let cool slightly before serving.

Nutrition:

Calories 153 Total Carbs 10g Net Carbs 5g Protein 9g Fat 8g Sugar 1g Fiber 5g

Seafood

14   Grilled Tuna Salad

Preparation time: 10 minutes

Cooking time: 30 minutes

Servings: 4

Ingredients:

4 oz. tuna fish, 4 steaks

¾ lb. red potatoes, diced

½ lb. green beans, trimmed

16 kalamata olives, chopped

4 cups of baby spinach leaves

What you will need from the store cupboard:

2 tablespoons canola oil

2 tablespoons red wine vinegar

1/8 teaspoon salt

1 tablespoon water

1/8 teaspoon red pepper flakes

Directions:

Steam the green beans and potatoes to make them tender.

Drain, rinse to shake off the excess water.

Bring together the vinaigrette ingredients in your jar while the vegetables are cooking. Close the lid and shake well. Everything should blend well.

Brush the vinaigrette over your fish.

Coat canola oil on your pan. Heat over medium temperature.

Grill each side of the tuna for 3 minutes.

Now divide the greens on your serving plates.

Arrange the green beans, olives, and potatoes over the greens.

Drizzle the vinaigrette on the salad. Top with tuna.

Nutrition: Calories 345, Carbohydrates 26g, Fiber 5g, Cholesterol 40mg, Total Fat 14g, Protein 29g, Sodium 280mg

15   Crab Curry

Preparation time: 10 minutes

Cooking time: 30 minutes

Servings: 2

Ingredients:

0.5lb chopped crab

1 thinly sliced red onion

0.5 cup chopped tomato

3tbsp curry paste

1tbsp oil or ghee

Directions:

Set the Instant Pot to saute and add the onion, oil, and curry paste.

When the onion is soft, add the remaining ingredients and seal.

Cook on Stew for 20 minutes.

Release the pressure naturally.

Nutrition: Calories: 250;Carbs: 11 ;Sugar: 4 ;Fat: 10 ;Protein: 24 ;GL: 9

16   Mussels And Spaghetti Squash

Preparation time: 10 minutes

Cooking time: 30 minutes

Servings: 2

Ingredients:

1lb cooked, shelled mussels

1/2 a spaghetti squash, to fit the Instant Pot

1 cup low sodium fish broth

3tbsp crushed garlic

sea salt to taste

Directions:

Mix the mussels with the garlic and salt. Place the mussels inside the squash.

Lower the squash into your Instant Pot.

Pour the broth around it, cook on Stew for 35 minutes.

Release the pressure naturally.

Shred the squash, mixing the "spaghetti" with the mussels.

Nutrition: Calories 265, Carbs 7g, Fat 9 g, Protein 24 g, Potassium (K) 124.8 mg, Sodium (Na) 462.6 mg

17   Shrimp With Tomatoes And Feta

Preparation time: 10 minutes

Cooking time: 30 minutes

Servings: 6

Ingredients:

2 tbsp. butter

1 lb. frozen shrimp

1 tbsp. garlic

1½ cups chopped white onion

14.5 oz. crushed tomatoes

1 tsp. dried oregano

1 tsp. sea salt

½ tsp. red pepper flakes, or to taste

To Serve:

1 cup crumbled feta cheese

½ cup sliced black olives

¼ cup fresh parsley

Directions:

Select the "Sauté" function on your Instant Pot and once hot, add the butter.

Melt the butter and then add the garlic and red pepper flakes.

Next, add in the onions, tomatoes, salt, and oregano.

Add the frozen shrimp.

Set the Instant pot on "Manual, High Pressure" setting for1 minute.

Once done, release all the pressure and stir well to combine all the ingredients.

Allow to cool and then sprinkle with feta cheese, black olives, and parsley.

Serve with buttered French bread, or rice.

Nutrition: Calories 211, Carbs 6g, Fat 11 g, Protein 19 g, Potassium (K) 148 mg, Sodium (Na) 1468 mg

18 Lemon Pepper And Dill Salmon

Preparation time: 10 minutes

Cooking time: 30 minutes

Servings: 4

Ingredients:

2 tbsp. butter

1 lb. salmon filet

1 sliced lemon

3 thyme sprigs

1 fresh dill sprig

1 tsp. chopped dill

Juice of 1 lemon

Zest of 1 lemon

1 tsp. sea salt

¼ tsp. black pepper

Directions:

Add the butter, lemon zest, lemon juice, dill, salt, and pepper to a small mixing bowl. Mix well to form a compound butter. Cut salmon into portion sizes, and place dollops of the compound butter all around the salmon portions.

Pour a cup of water into the Instant Pot, along with some thyme and/or dill.

Place half of the salmon onto a standard trivet and insert this into the pot.

Season with more pepper, and then top the fish with 2 thin slices of lemon.

Place the second half of the fish onto a 3-inch trivet and insert into the pot. Season with more black pepper, and then top the salmon again with 2 thin slices of lemon.

Close and lock the lid, cooking on "Manual, High Pressure" for 3 minutes.

Once done, quick release the pressure.

Uncover, and serve immediately.

Nutrition: Calories 224, Carbs 3g, Fat 13g, Protein 22 g, Potassium (K) 602 mg, Sodium (Na) 581 mg

Poultry

19   Chicken With Cashew Nuts

Preparation time: 10 minutes

Cooking time: 30 minutes

Servings: 4

Ingredients:

1 lb chicken cubes

2 tbsp soy sauce

1 tbsp corn flour

2 ½ onion cubes

1 carrot, chopped

⅓ cup cashew nuts, fried

1 capsicum, cut

2 tbsp garlic, crushed

Salt and white pepper

Directions:

Marinate the chicken cubes with ½ tbsp of white pepper, ½ tsp salt, 2 tbsp soya sauce, and add 1 tbsp corn flour.
Set aside for 25 minutes. Preheat the Air Fryer to 380 F and transfer the marinated chicken. Add the garlic, the onion, the capsicum, and the carrot; fry for 5-6 minutes. Roll it in the cashew nuts before serving.

Nutrition: Calories: 425; Carbs: 25gFat: 35gProtein: 53g

20 Chuck And Veggies

Preparation time: 10 minutes

Cooking time: 30 minutes

Servings: 2

Ingredients:

¼ cup dry red wine

¼ teaspoon salt

8 oz. boneless lean chuck roast

¼ teaspoon black pepper

8 oz. frozen pepper stir-fry

1 teaspoon Worcestershire sauce

8 oz. whole mushrooms

1 teaspoon instant coffee granules

1 1/4 cups fresh green beans, trimmed

1 dried bay leaf

Directions:

Mix all the ingredients except salt in a bowl; combine well and then transfer to a slow cooker.

Cover the cooker and cook for about 9 hours on low and 4 1/2 hours on high, until beef is completely cooked through and tender.

Stir in ¼ teaspoon salt gently. Take out the vegetables and beef and transfer to 2 shallow bowls.

Pour liquid into the skillet; boil it lightly and cook until liquid reduces to ¼ cup, for about 1 1/2 minutes.

Pour over veggies and beef. Discard bay leaf and serve.

Nutrition: 215 calories; 5 g fat; 17 g total carbs; 26 g protein

21 Chicken & Broccoli Bake

Preparation time: 10 minutes

Cooking time: 30 minutes

Servings: 6

Ingredients:

6 (6-ounce) boneless, skinless chicken breasts

3 broccoli heads, cut into florets

4 garlic cloves, minced

¼ cup olive oil

1 teaspoon dried oregano, crushed

1 teaspoon dried rosemary, crushed

Sea Salt and ground black pepper, as required

Directions:

Preheat the oven to 375 degrees F. Grease a large baking dish.

In a large bowl, add all the ingredients and toss to coat well.

In the bottom of prepared baking dish, arrange the broccoli florets and top with chicken breasts in a single layer.

Bake for about 45 minutes.

Remove from the oven and set aside for about 5 minutes before serving.

Meal Prep Tip: Remove the baking dish from the oven and set aside to cool completely. In 6 containers, divide the chicken breasts and broccoli evenly and refrigerate for about 2 days. Reheat in microwave before serving.

Nutrition: Calories 443 Total Fat 21.5 g Saturated Fat 4.7 g Cholesterol 151 mg Total Carbs 9.4 g Sugar 2.2g Fiber 3.6 g Sodium 189 mg Potassium 831 mg Protein 53 g

22   Hoisin Chicken Lettuce Wraps

Preparation time: 10 minutes

Cooking time: 30 minutes

Servings: 4

Ingredients:

For the chicken

2 teaspoons peanut oil

⅓ cup low-sodium gluten-free tamari or soy sauce

1 tablespoon honey

2 tablespoons rice vinegar

2 teaspoons Sriracha sauce

1 tablespoon minced garlic

2 teaspoons peeled and minced fresh ginger

⅓ cup Chicken Bone Broth or water

2 scallions, both white and green parts, thinly sliced, divided

1 bone-in, skin-on chicken breast (about 1 pound)

For the lettuce wraps

Large lettuce leaves (preferably Bibb)

1 cup broccoli slaw or shredded cabbage

¼ cup chopped cashews, toasted

Directions:

To make the chicken

In the electric pressure cooker, whisk together the peanut oil, tamari, honey, rice vinegar, Sriracha, garlic, ginger, and broth. Stir in the white parts of the scallions.

Place the chicken breast in the sauce, meat-side down.

Close and lock the lid of the pressure cooker. Set the valve to sealing.

Cook on high pressure for 20 minutes.

When the cooking is complete, hit Cancel and quick release the pressure.

Once the pin drops, unlock and remove the lid.

Using tongs, transfer the chicken breast to a cutting board.

When the chicken is cool enough to handle, remove the skin, shred the chicken, and return it to the pot. Let the chicken soak in the sauce for at least 5 minutes.

To make the lettuce wraps

Spoon some of the chicken and sauce into the lettuce leaves.

Sprinkle with the broccoli slaw, the green parts of the scallions, and the cashews.

Serve immediately.

Nutrition: Calories: 233; Total Fat: 13gProtein: 14gCarbohydrates: 18gSugars: 10gFiber: 2gSodium: 1080mg

23   Zucchini With Tomatoes

Preparation time: 10 minutes

Cooking time: 30 minutes

Servings: 8

Ingredients:

6 medium zucchinis, chopped roughly

1 pound cherry tomatoes

2 small onions, chopped roughly

2 tablespoons fresh basil, chopped

1 cup water

1 tablespoon olive oil

2 garlic cloves, minced

Salt and ground black pepper, as required

Directions:

In the Instant Pot, place oil and press "Sauté". Now add the onion, garlic, ginger, and spices and cook for about 3-4 minutes.

Add the zucchinis and tomatoes and cook for about 1-2 minutes.

Press "Cancel" and stir in the remaining ingredients except basil.

Close the lid and place the pressure valve to "Seal" position.

Press "Manual" and cook under "High Pressure" for about 5 minutes.

Press "Cancel" and allow a "Natural" release.

Open the lid and transfer the vegetable mixture onto a serving platter.

Garnish with basil and serve.

Nutrition: Calories: 57, Fats: 2.1g, Carbs: 9g, Sugar: 4.8g, Proteins: 2.5g, Sodium: 39mg

24   Chicken Liver Curry

Preparation time: 10 minutes

Cooking time: 30 minutes

Servings: 2

Ingredients:

1lb diced chicken breast

0.5lb diced chicken liver

1lb chopped vegetables

1 cup broth

3tbsp curry paste

Directions:

Mix all the ingredients in your Instant Pot.

Cook on Stew for 35 minutes.

Release the pressure naturally.

Nutrition: Calories: 350;Carbs: 10 ;Sugar: 2 ;Fat: 17 ;Protein: 52 ;GL: 4

Soup and Stews

25   Chipotle Chicken & Corn Soup

Preparation time: 15 minutes

Cooking time: 30 minutes

Servings: 8

Ingredients:

1 onion, diced

2 chipotle peppers in adobo sauce, diced

3 cup corn kernels

2 cup chicken breast, cooked and cut in cubes

½ cup fat free sour cream

¼ cup cilantro, diced

What you'll need from store cupboard:

2 14 ½ oz. cans fire roasted tomatoes, diced

4 cup low sodium chicken broth

4 cloves garlic, diced

1 tbsp. sunflower oil

2 tsp adobo sauce

1 tsp cumin

¼ tsp pepper

Directions:

Heat oil in a large pot over med-high heat. Add onion and cook until tender, about 3-5 minutes. Add garlic and cook 1 minute more.

Add broth, tomatoes, corn, chipotle peppers, adobo sauce, and seasonings. Bring to a boil. Reduce heat and simmer 20 minutes.

Stir in chicken and cook until heated through. Serve garnished with sour cream and cilantro.

Nutrition:

Calories 145 Total Carbs 20g Net Carbs 16g Protein 10g Fat 3g Sugar 6g Fiber 4g

26   Chorizo & Corn Chowder

Preparation time: 15 minutes

Cooking time: 4 ½ hours

Servings: 4

Ingredients:

1 onion, diced

1 fennel bulb, cut in ¼-inch pieces

6 sprigs fresh thyme

3 oz. cured chorizo

2 cup cauliflower, separate in small florets

1 ½ cup corn, frozen

½ cup half-n-half

What you'll need from store cupboard:

4 cup low sodium chicken broth

2 cloves garlic, diced fine

2 tbsp. flour

Salt & pepper, to taste

Directions:

Place cauliflower, onion, fennel, corn, garlic, and half the chorizo in a crock pot. Stir in flour and ½ teaspoon each salt and pepper.

Pour in the broth and thyme and stir to combine. Cover and cook on high heat 4 ½ hours, or until vegetables are tender.

Ten minutes before serving, add remaining chorizo to a hot skillet and cook over med-high heat until browned and crisp, about 3 minutes.

Discard the thyme and stir in half-n-half. Ladle into bowls and garnish with chorizo.

Nutrition:

Calories 206 Total Carbs 26g Net Carbs 21g Protein 12g Fat 7g Sugar 5g Fiber 5g

27   Chunky Chicken Noodle Soup

Preparation time: 10 minutes

Cooking time 35 minutes

Servings: 8

Ingredients:

2 lbs. chicken thighs, boneless and skinless

2 carrots, sliced

2 celery stalks, sliced

2 tsp fresh ginger, grated

What you'll need from store cupboard:

8 cup low sodium chicken broth

2 cup homemade pasta

1 tbsp. garlic, diced fine

1 tbsp. chicken bouillon

Salt and pepper, to taste

Directions:

Place chicken and 1 cup broth in a large soup pot over medium heat. Bring to a simmer and cook until chicken is done, about 20 minutes. Transfer chicken to a bowl and shred using 2 forks.

Add the carrots, celery, garlic, ginger, and bouillon to the pot and stir well. Add in remaining broth and bring back to a boil. Reduce heat and simmer until vegetables are tender, about 15 minutes.

Add pasta and cook another 5 minutes for fresh pasta, or 7 for dried. Add the chicken to the soup and salt and pepper to taste. Serve.

Nutrition:

Calories 210 Total Carbs 15g Net Carbs 12g Protein 23g Fat 7g Sugar 7g Fiber 3g

28   Cioppino

Preparation time: 20 minutes

Cooking time: 45 minutes

Servings: 6

Ingredients:

20 hard shelled clams

20 shelled mussels

1 lb. red snapper

1 lb. very large shrimp, deveined, shell-on

1 lb. large sea scallops, muscles removed from side if attached

3 stalks celery, sliced thin

2 onions, diced fine

1 yellow pepper, seeded and diced

¼ cup fresh parsley, chopped

¼ cup fresh basil, chopped

What you'll need from store cupboard

1 can whole plum tomatoes, drained and chopped, reserve juice

1 ½ cup dry white wine

1 cup bottled clam juice

1 cup low sodium chicken broth

¼ cup light olive oil

8 cloves garlic, diced fine

2 tbsp. tomato paste

2 tbsp. Splenda

2 bay leaves

1 ½ tsp salt

1 tsp black pepper

1 tsp oregano

Directions:

Add onion, oil, garlic, bay leaves, oregano, salt and pepper to a large pot and cook over medium heat until onions are soft. Stir in celery, bell pepper, and tomato paste and cook, stirring, 1 minute. Add wine and bring to a boil, cook until liquid is reduced by half, about 5-6 minutes.

Stir in tomatoes, reserved juice, clam juice, broth and Splenda. Reduce heat and simmer, covered 30 minutes.

Add the clams and mussels and cook until they open. Transfer opened clams and mussels to a bowl as soon as they open. Discard any that do not open.

Season fish, shrimp and scallops with salt and pepper and add to the pot. Simmer covered 3 minutes or just until shrimp start to turn pink. If shrimp cooks before the fish, remove it to a bowl.

Turn off heat and discard bay leaves. Return all cooked seafood back to the pot and add parsley. Serve warm garnished with chopped basil.

Nutrition:

Calories 514 Total Carbs 26g Net Carbs 23g Protein 62g Fat 13g Sugar 13g Fiber 3g

29   Clam & Bacon Soup

Preparation time: 20 minutes

Cooking time: 20 minutes

Servings: 8

Ingredients:

10-12 large clams, in the shell

4 slices bacon, chopped and cooked almost crisp

3 cups cauliflower, separated into florets

½ cup onion, diced

What you'll need from store cupboard:

6 cup water

1 tsp Worcestershire sauce

Directions:

Scrub clams and rinse under cold running water. Place in a large pot and add water. Bring to a simmer over med-high heat. Cover and cook until clams open, about 8-10 minutes. Transfer clams to bowl to cool.

Cook onion in the same pan used for the bacon, 2-3 minutes. Stir to scrape up the brown bits on the bottom of the pan. When clams are cool enough to touch, remove the meat from the shells and chop it.

Bring the clam liquid to a boil. Add cauliflower and cook until almost tender, about 5 minutes.

Stir in the bacon, Worcestershire sauce and clams. Season with salt and pepper to taste and cook until everything is heated through. Serve immediately.

Nutrition:

Calories 105 Total Carbs 4g Protein 7g Fat 7g Sugar 2g Fiber 1g

30   Crab & Cauliflower Bisque

Preparation time: 20 minutes

Cooking time: 30 minutes

Servings: 8

Ingredients:

1 lb. lump crabmeat, cooked and shells removed

1 medium head cauliflower, separated into very small florets

1 white onion, diced fine

1 cup celery, diced fine

1 cup carrots, diced fine

1 cup half-n-half

1 tbsp. sherry

4 tbsp. margarine

What you'll need from store cupboard:

6 cup chicken broth

1½ tsp coarse salt

1 tsp white pepper

Directions:

In a large saucepan, over med-high heat, melt margarine. Add celery, onion, and carrot. Cook, stirring frequently, until vegetables are tender.

Add in cauliflower, broth, salt, and pepper, and cook until soup starts to boil. Reduce heat to medium and cook 15 minutes, or until cauliflower is tender.

Pour into a blender and add cream and sherry. Process until combined and soup is smooth. Pour back into the saucepan. Fold in crab and heat through. Serve.

Nutrition:

Calories 201 Total Carbs 10g Net Carbs 7g Protein 14g Fat 11g Sugar 4g Fiber 3g

31   Creamy Chicken & Cauliflower Rice Soup

Preparation time: 20 minutes

Cooking time: 5 hours

Servings: 6

Ingredients:

2 carrots, peeled and diced

2 stalks celery, peeled and diced

1/2 onion, diced

2 cup skim milk

2 cups cauliflower, riced

1 cup chicken, cooked and shredded

3 tbsp. Margarine

What you'll need from store cupboard:

4 cup low sodium chicken broth

5 cloves garlic, diced

½ tsp rosemary

½ tsp thyme

½ tsp parsley

1 bay leaf

Directions:

Melt margarine in a large skillet over medium heat. Add carrots, celery, onion and garlic. Cook, stirring frequently, about 5 minutes. Place in crock pot.

Add chicken broth and seasonings. Cover and cook on low 4 hours.

Add in the chicken, milk and cauliflower rice. Cook another 60 minutes or until cauliflower is tender. Discard bay leaf before serving.

Nutrition:

Calories 151 Total Carbs 10g Net Carbs 8g Protein 12g Fat 6g Sugar 6g Fiber 2g

32. Creamy Sweet Potato & Cauliflower Bisque

Preparation time: 10 minutes

Cooking time: 20 minutes

Servings: 4

Ingredients:

1 head cauliflower, separated into large florets

1 large sweet potato, peeled and cut into cubes

1 onion, diced fine

1 cup skim milk

1/3 block of low fat cream cheese, cut into cubes

1 tsp margarine

What you'll need from store cupboard:

2 cup low sodium vegetable broth

2 cloves garlic, peeled

½ tsp rosemary

1/8 tsp red pepper flakes

Salt and pepper to taste

Directions:

Melt margarine in a large sauce pan over med-high heat. Add onion, and cook until soft, 2-3 minutes.

Add remaining vegetables, broth and seasonings and bring to a boil. Reduce heat to low and cook until potato is soft, 12-15 minutes.

Stir in the milk and cream cheese until cheese has melted. Use an immersion blender and process until smooth. Taste and add salt and pepper if needed. Serve.

Nutrition:

Calories 125 Total Carbs 23g Net Carbs 18g Protein 9g Fat 0g Sugar 10g Fiber 5g

33   Curried Chicken Soup

Preparation time: 15 minutes

Cooking time: 20 minutes

Servings: 12

Ingredients:

2 carrots, diced

2 stalks celery, diced

1 onion, diced

3 cup chicken, cooked and cut in cubes

2 cups cauliflower, grated

1 cup half-n-half

¼ cup margarine, cubed

What you'll need from store cupboard:

4 ½ cup low sodium vegetable broth

2 12 oz. can fat free evaporated milk

¾ cup + 2 tbsp. flour

1 tsp salt

1 tsp curry powder

Directions:

Melt butter in a large pot over medium heat. Add carrots, celery, and onion and cook 2 minutes.

Stir in flour until well blended. Stir in seasonings. Slowly add milk and half-n-half. Bring to a boil, cook, stirring, 2 minutes or until thickened.

Slowly stir in broth. Add chicken and cauliflower and bring back to boil. Reduce heat and simmer 10 minutes, or until vegetable are tender. Serve.

Nutrition:

Calories 204 Total Carbs 17g Protein 17g Fat 7g Sugar 8g Fiber 1g

---

Salads, Sauces, Dressings & Dips

34   Parmesan-Topped Acorn Squash

Preparation Time: 8 minutes

Cooking Time: 20 minutes

Servings: 4

Ingredients:

1 acorn squash (about 1 pound)

1 tablespoon extra-virgin olive oil

1 teaspoon dried sage leaves, crumbled

¼ teaspoon freshly grated nutmeg

1/8 teaspoon kosher salt

1/8 teaspoon freshly ground black pepper

2 tablespoons freshly grated Parmesan cheese

Directions:

1. Chop acorn squash in half lengthwise and remove the seeds. Cut each half in half for a total of 4 wedges. Snap off the stem if it's easy to do.

2. In a small bowl, combine the olive oil, sage, nutmeg, salt, and pepper. Brush the cut sides of the squash with the olive oil mixture.

3. Fill 1 cup of water into the electric pressure cooker and insert a wire rack or trivet.

4. Place the squash on the trivet in a single layer, skin-side down.

5. Set the lid of the pressure cooker on sealing.

6. Cook on high pressure for 20 minutes.

7. Once done, press Cancel and quick release the pressure.

8. Once the pin drops, open it.

9. Carefully remove the squash from the pot, sprinkle with the Parmesan, and serve.

Nutrition:

85 Calories

12g Carbohydrates

2g Fiber

35   Quinoa Tabbouleh

Preparation Time: 8 minutes

Cooking Time: 16 minutes

Servings: 6

Ingredients:

1 cup quinoa, rinsed

1 large English cucumber

2 scallions, sliced

2 cups cherry tomatoes, halved

2/3 cup chopped parsley

1/2 cup chopped mint

½ teaspoon minced garlic

1/2 teaspoon salt

½ teaspoon ground black pepper

2 tablespoon lemon juice

1/2 cup olive oil

Directions:

1. Plugin instant pot, insert the inner pot, add quinoa, then pour in water and stir until mixed.

2. Close instant pot with its lid and turn the pressure knob to seal the pot.

3. Select 'manual' button, then set the 'timer' to 1 minute and cook in high pressure, it may take 7 minutes.

4. Once the timer stops, select 'cancel' button and do natural pressure release for 10 minutes and then do quick pressure release until pressure nob drops down.

5. Open the instant pot, fluff quinoa with a fork, then spoon it on a rimmed baking sheet, spread quinoa evenly and let cool.

6. Meanwhile, place lime juice in a small bowl, add garlic and stir until just mixed.

7. Then add salt, black pepper, and olive oil and whisk until combined.

8. Transfer cooled quinoa to a large bowl, add remaining ingredients, then drizzle generously with the prepared lime juice mixture and toss until evenly coated.

9. Taste quinoa to adjust seasoning and then serve.

Nutrition:

283 Calories

30.6g Carbohydrates

3.4g Fiber

36   Wild Rice Salad with Cranberries and Almonds

Preparation Time: 6 minutes

Cooking Time: 25 minutes

Servings: 18

Ingredients:

For the rice

2 cups wild rice blend, rinsed

1 teaspoon kosher salt

2½ cups Vegetable Broth

For the dressing

¼ cup extra-virgin olive oil

¼ cup white wine vinegar

1½ teaspoons grated orange zest

Juice of 1 medium orange (about ¼ cup)

1 teaspoon honey or pure maple syrup

For the salad

¾ cup unsweetened dried cranberries

½ cup sliced almonds, toasted

Freshly ground black pepper

Directions:

1. To make the rice 2. In the electric pressure cooker, combine the rice, salt, and broth.

3. Close and lock the lid. Set the valve to sealing.

4. Cook on high pressure for 25 minutes.

5. When the cooking is complete, hit Cancel and allow the pressure to release naturally for 1minutes, then quick release any remaining pressure.

6. Once the pin drops, unlock and remove the lid.

7. Let the rice cool briefly, then fluff it with a fork.

8. To make the dressing 9. While the rice cooks, make the dressing: In a small jar with a screw-top lid, combine the olive oil, vinegar, zest, juice, and honey. (If you don't have a jar, whisk the ingredients together in a small bowl.) Shake to combine.

10. To make the salad 11. Mix rice, cranberries, and almonds.

12. Add the dressing and season with pepper.

13. Serve warm or refrigerate.

Nutrition

126 Calories

18g Carbohydrates

2g Fiber

37 Low Fat Roasties

Preparation Time: 8 minutes

Cooking Time: 25 minutes

Servings: 2

Ingredients:

1lb roasting potatoes

1 garlic clove

1 cup vegetable stock

2tbsp olive oil

Directions:

1. Position potatoes in the steamer basket and add the stock into the Instant Pot.

2. Steam the potatoes in your Instant Pot for 15 minutes.

3. Depressurize and pour away the remaining stock.

4. Set to sauté and add the oil, garlic, and potatoes. Cook until brown.

Nutrition:

201 Calories

3g Carbohydrates

6g Fat

Dessert and Snacks

38   Green Fruity Smoothie

Preparation time: 10 minutes

Cooking time: 30 minutes

Servings: 2

Cooking Time: 10 Minutes

Ingredients:

1 cup frozen mango, peeled, pitted, and chopped

1 large frozen banana, peeled

2 cups fresh baby spinach

1 scoop unsweetened vegan vanilla protein powder

¼ cup pumpkin seeds

2 tablespoons hemp hearts

1½ cups unsweetened almond milk

Directions:

In a high-speed blender, place all the ingredients and pulse until creamy.

Pour into two glasses and serve immediately.

Nutrition: Calories 355 Total Fat 16.1 g Saturated Fat 2.4 g Cholesterol 0 mg Sodium 295 mg Total Carbs 34.6 g Fiber 6.2 g Sugar 19.9 g Protein 23.4 g

39   Baked Creamy Custard With Maple

Preparation time: 10 minutes

Cooking time: 30 minutes

Servings: 6

Ingredients:

2 1/2 cups half-and-half, fat-free

1/2 cup egg substitute, cholesterol-free

1/4 cup sugar

2 teaspoons vanilla

Dash ground nutmeg

3 cups of boiling water

2 tablespoons of maple syrup

Directions:

Spray 6 ramekins or custard cups with light nonstick cooking spray. Preheat your oven to 325°F.

Combine first five ingredients and mix well. Pour into your ramekins.

Pour the boiling water in a 13x9-inch baking dish. Place the ramekins in the dish and bake 1 hour 15 minutes.

Cool the ramekins on a cooling rack. Cover with a plastic wrap and chill in the fridge overnight.

Drizzle with maple syrup before serving.

Nutrition: Calories: 131 Carbohydrates: 23 g Fiber: 0 g Fats: 1 g Sodium: 139 mg Protein: 5 g

40   Lemon Cookies

Preparation time: 10 minutes

Cooking time: 30 minutes

Servings: 6

Ingredients:

¼ cup unsweetened applesauce

1 cup cashew butter

1 teaspoon fresh lemon zest, grated finely

2 tablespoons fresh lemon juice

Pinch of sea salt

Directions:

Preheat the oven to 350 degrees F. Line a large cookie sheet with parchment paper.

In a food processor, add all ingredients and pulse until smooth.

With a tablespoon, place the mixture onto prepared cookie sheet in a single layer.

Bake for about 12 minutes or until golden brown.

Remove from oven and place the cookie sheet onto a wire rack to cool for about 5 minutes.

Carefully invert the cookies onto wire rack to cool completely before serving.

Meal Prep Tip: Store these cookies in an airtight container, by placing parchment papers between the cookies to avoid the sticking. These cookies can be stored in the refrigerator for up to 2 weeks.

Nutrition: Calories 257 Total Fat 21.9 g Saturated Fat 4.2 g Cholesterol 0 mg Total Carbs 13.1 g Sugar 1.2 g Fiber 1 g Sodium 47 mg Potassium 248 mg Protein 7.6 g

41   Pineapple Nice Cream

Preparation time: 10 minutes

Cooking time: 30 minutes

Servings: 6

Ingredients:

1 16-oz. package frozen pineapple chunks

1 cup frozen mango chunks or 1 large mango, peeled, seeded and chopped

1 tbsp. lemon juice or lime juice

Directions:

In a food processor, process the mango, lemon or lime juice, and pineapple until creamy and smooth. You can add a 1/4 cup of water if the mango is frozen. Serve it immediately if you want to have the best texture.

Nutrition: Calories: 55 calories; Total Carbohydrate: 14 g Cholesterol: 0 mg Total Fat: 0 g Fiber: 2 g Protein: 1 g Sodium: 1 mg Sugar: 11 g Saturated Fat: 0 g

42   Garden Salad Wraps

Preparation time: 10 minutes

Cooking time: 30 minutes

Servings: 4

Ingredients:

6 tablespoons extra-virgin olive oil

1-pound extra-firm tofu, drained, patted dry, and cut into ½-inch strips

1 tablespoon soy sauce

¼ cup apple cider vinegar

1 teaspoon yellow or spicy brown mustard

½ teaspoon salt

¼ teaspoon freshly ground black pepper

3 cups shredded romaine lettuce

3 ripe Roma tomatoes, finely chopped

1 large carrot, shredded

1 medium English cucumber, peeled and chopped

⅓ cup minced red onion

¼ cup sliced pitted green olives

4 (10-inch) whole-grain flour tortillas or lavish flatbread

Directions:

Preparing the Ingredients

Cook the tofu until golden brown in a large skillet with Over medium heat. Sprinkle with soy sauce and set aside to cool.

In a small bowl, combine the vinegar, mustard, salt and pepper with the remaining 4 tablespoons oil, stirring to blend well. Set aside.

Finish and Serve

combine the cucumber, onion, lettuce, tomatoes, carrot, and olives in a large bowl. Pour on the dressing.

Put 1 tortilla on a work surface and spread with about one-quarter of the salad. Place a few strips of tofu on the tortilla and roll up tightly. Slice in half.

Nutrition: 191 Cal 16.6 g Fats 9.6 g Protein 0.8 g Net Carb 0.2 g Fiber

43   Berry Mint Smoothie

Preparation Time: 5 Minutes

Cooking Time: 5 Minutes

Servings: 2

Ingredients:

1 tbsp. Low-carb Sweetener of your choice

1 cup Kefir or Low Fat-Yoghurt

2 tbsp. Mint

¼ cup Orange

1 cup Mixed Berries

Directions:

Place all the ingredients needed to make the smoothie in a high-speed blender and blend until smooth.

Transfer the smoothie to a serving glass and enjoy it.

Tip: You can add flax seeds or chia seeds if you prefer to make it more nutritious.

Nutrition: Calories: 137Kcal Carbohydrates: 11g Proteins: 6g Fat: 1g Sodium: 64mg

44   Greenie Smoothie

Preparation Time: 5 Minutes

Cooking Time: 5 Minutes

Servings: 2

Ingredients:

1 ½ cup Water

1 tsp. Stevia

1 Green Apple, ripe

1 tsp. Stevia

1 Green Pear, chopped into chunks

1 Lime

2 cups Kale, fresh

¾ tsp. Cinnamon

12 Ice Cubes

20 Green Grapes

½ cup Mint, fresh

Directions:

Pour water, kale, and pear in a high-speed blender and blend them for 2 to 3 minutes until mixed.

Stir in all the remaining ingredients into it and blend until it becomes smooth.

Transfer the smoothie to serving glass.

Tip: You can stir in a teaspoon of stevia if needed.

Nutrition: Calories: 123Kcal Carbohydrates: 27g Proteins: 2g Fat: 2g Sodium: 30mg

45   Coconut Spinach Smoothie

Preparation Time: 5 Minutes

Cooking Time: 0 Minutes

Servings: 2

Ingredients:

1 ¼ cup Coconut Milk

2 Ice Cubes

2 tbsp. Chia Seeds

1 scoop of Protein Powder, preferably vanilla

1 cup Spin

Directions:

Pour coconut milk along with spinach, chia seeds, protein powder, and ice cubes in a high-speed blender.

Blend for 2 minutes to get a smooth and luscious smoothie.

Serve in a glass and enjoy it.

Tip: You can avoid protein powder if not desired.

Nutrition: Calories: 251Kcal Carbohydrates: 10.9g Proteins: 20.3g Fat: 15.1g Sodium: 102mg

46   Oats Coffee Smoothie

Preparation Time: 5 Minutes

Cooking Time: 5 Minutes

Servings: 2

Ingredients:

1 cup Oats, uncooked & grounded

2 tbsp. Instant Coffee

3 cup Milk, skimmed

2 Banana, frozen & sliced into chunks

2 tbsp. Flax Seeds, grounded

Directions:

Place all the ingredients in a high-speed blender and blend for 2 minutes or until smooth and luscious.

Serve and enjoy.

Tip: If you need more sweetness, one teaspoon of any low-carb sweetener.

Nutrition: Calories: 251Kcal Carbohydrates: 10.9g Proteins: 20.3g Fat: 15.1g Sodium: 102mg

47   Avocado Smoothie

Preparation Time: 10 Minutes

Cooking Time: 0 Minutes

Servings: 2

Ingredients:

1 Avocado, ripe & pit removed

2 cups Baby Spinach

2 cups Water

1 cup Baby Kale

1 tbsp. Lemon Juice

2 sprigs of Mint

½ cup Ice Cubes

Directions:

Place all the ingredients needed to make the smoothie in a high-speed blender and blend until smooth.

Transfer to a serving glass and enjoy it.

Tip: If you want to add more sweetness, you can add a pinch of honey.

Nutrition: Calories: 214cal Carbohydrates: 15g Proteins: 2g Fat: 17g Sodium: 25mg

48   Orange Carrot Smoothie

Preparation Time: 5 Minutes

Cooking Time: 0 Minutes

Servings: 1

Ingredients:

1 ½ cups Almond Milk

¼ cup Cauliflower, blanched & frozen

1 Orange

1 tbsp. Flax Seed

1/3 cup Carrot, grated

1 tsp. Vanilla Extract

Directions:

Mix all the ingredients in a high-speed blender and blend for 2 minutes or until you get the desired consistency.

Transfer to a serving glass and enjoy it.

Tip: If you want to make it more nutritious, you can add collagen powder.

Nutrition: Calories: 216cal Carbohydrates: 10g Proteins: 15g Fat: 7g Sodium: 25mg

49   Blackberry Smoothie

Preparation Time: 5 Minutes

Cooking Time: 0 Minutes

Servings: 1

Ingredients:

1 ½ cups Almond Milk

¼ cup Cauliflower, blanched & frozen

1 Orange

1 tbsp. Flax Seed

1/3 cup Carrot, grated

1 tsp. Vanilla Extract

Directions:

Place all the ingredients needed to make the blackberry smoothie in a high-speed blender and blend for 2 minutes until you get a smooth mixture.

Transfer to a serving glass and enjoy it.

Tip: Instead of cauliflower, you can also use blanched & frozen zucchini.

Nutrition: Calories: 275cal Carbohydrates: 9g Proteins: 11g Fat: 17g Sodium: 73mg

50   Key Lime Pie Smoothie

Preparation Time: 5 Minutes

Cooking Time: 0 Minutes

Servings: 1

Ingredients:

½ cup Cottage Cheese

1 tbsp. Sweetener of your choice

½ cup Water

½ cup Spinach

1 tbsp. Lime Juice

1 cup Ice Cubes

Directions:

Spoon in the ingredients to a high-speed blender and blend until silky smooth.

Transfer to a serving glass and enjoy it.

Tip: Instead of water, you can use almond milk to make it more nutritious and creamier.

Nutrition: Calories: 180cal Carbohydrates: 7g Proteins: 36g Fat: 1g Sodium: 35mg

Conclusion

Some years back, when someone got diagnosed with diabetes and was advised on diabetes diet, most would feel that they have been denied tasty food and would dislike the many restrictions that would come with such a diet. What such people did not realize is that they were switching to a healthier lifestyle. Today, most people are usually ready to take advice on diabetes diet and not feel that the restrictions are unnecessary.

Something that we need to get straight here is that diet for diabetic is a diet without harmful ingredients not without FLAVOR. In the past, diabetes diets were actually without flavor and this could be the major reason why most people disliked them. That has since changed and the diets available today from a dietician are as pleasant as any other meal would be. So if you were one of those people that had a negative connotation about diabetes diets due to taste, you should be changing that mentality now.

The benefits of a healthy diet for a diabetic are clear to many people today. However, it is important that we look at some of the benefits that most people may not have known. First, a diabetes diet is designed to keep your blood sugar at the recommended levels, not necessarily to reduce the blood sugar levels. If the glucose level in your blood falls below the recommended level, then it also becomes a problem.

When one is first diagnosed with diabetes, they have to start on medication immediately as they also embark on a healthy diet. After some time, if the patient observes a healthy diet strictly, it can be possible to reduce the amount of medication they need to take considerably. This is a major benefit of a diabetes diet.

In the end I would conclude with the fact that diabetes can at times develop as a result of being overweight. A good diet will not only help the patient's body regulate the blood sugar but also help them lose weight. A healthy weight is desirable to everyone, not only diabetics.